THE BEST OF *HEATH*

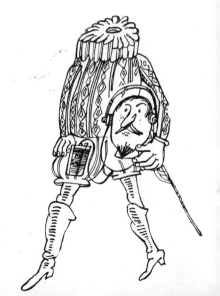

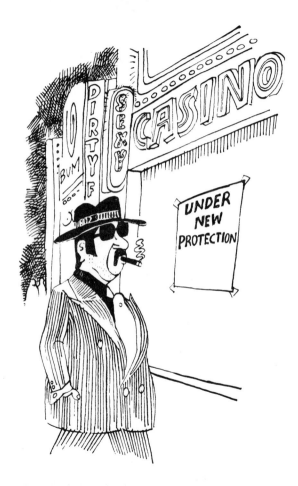

THE
BEST
OF

HEATH

Foreword by Malcolm Muggeridge

DAVID & CHARLES
Newton Abbot   London   North Pomfret

Heath and the publishers wish to thank the Editors of *Punch* and the *Spectator* for permission to use material from those magazines.

British Library Cataloguing in Publication Data

Heath, Michael
    The best of Heath.
    1. English wit and humour, Pictorial
    I. Title
    741.5'942   NC1479

    ISBN 0-7153-8601-8

Printed in Great Britain
by Redwood Burn Limited, Trowbridge, Wilts
for David & Charles (Publishers) Limited
Brunel House   Newton Abbot   Devon

Published in the United States of America
by David & Charles Inc
North Pomfret   Vermont 05053   USA

Foreword

Ever since I was editor of *Punch*, now some thirty years ago, I have taken an interest in small line drawings with a sharply worded caption. My attention was drawn to Heath's offerings in this vein by a joke of his about myself – Saint Peter has climbed up his ladder to Heaven to make his routine report to God, among other things mentioning that Mr M is again pestering for his release from mortality, and asking for a celestial *laisser passer*. To which God replies: 'Tell Mr M he must wait his turn like everyone else.'

Somehow, a joke about oneself is a special kind of compliment, even if, perhaps particularly if, it has a sting in it. Heath is adept at matching sharp words to sharp drawings; Ariel to his political namesake's Prospero. Thus a collection of his topical drawings provides a lively and useful record of the immediate past more memorable and entertaining than just words. A burst of laughter helps the past along, cuts down to size the demagogues of yesteryear, and brings the Churchills into line with the Attlees and the Humes, not to mention the Thatchers.

I once had an interesting conversation with the editorial staff of *Krokodil*, the only ostensibly satirical magazine published in the USSR. It was during the Khrushchev era, and I pointed out to my hosts that they had the inestimable advantage of a head man with a funny face, but made no use of it, whereas we on *Punch* had to make do with Harold Macmillan. They offered no comment.

Laughter is indeed inimical to power; Shakespeare's King John speaks of 'that idiot laughter . . . a passion hateful to my purposes', thereby speaking on behalf of all power maniacs, of whom we have seen a goodly crop in our time. A Heath helps to keep the laughter going, God bless him.

Malcolm Muggeridge

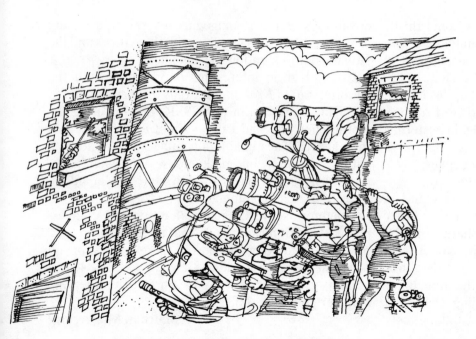

"I can't come out—I've got stage fright!"

"I had no idea that freeloading was a sin!"

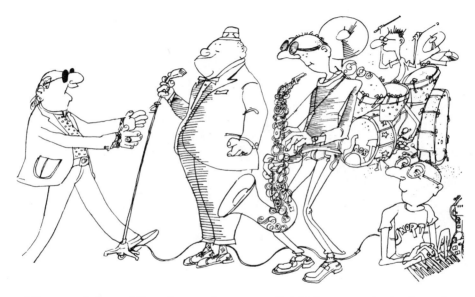

"*Congratulations, fellas—last week you were finished, now you're back on the nostalgia bandwagon.*"

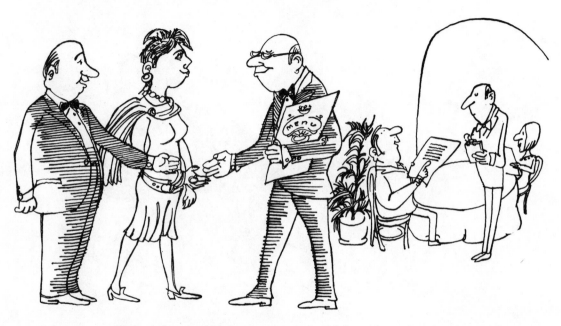

"I don't know what the restaurant would do without Gaston—he whips up the most wonderfully imaginative bills."

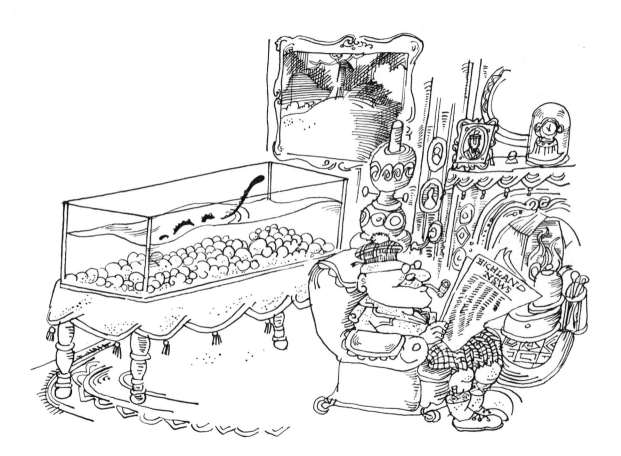

A spot of bovver

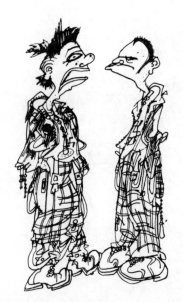

"I have a recurring nightmare that we've been accepted by society."

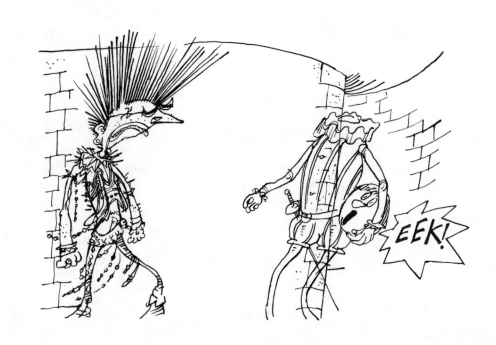

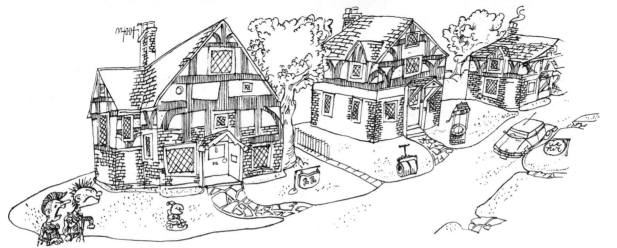

*"It's not a street I'd care to
walk down at night."*

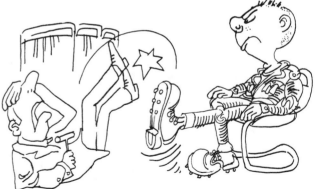

"Well, your reflexes are A.1."

A spot of bovver

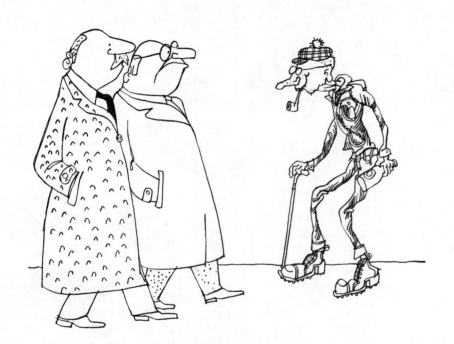

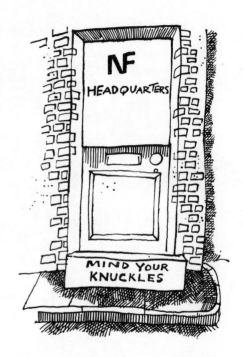

"*He's the local bowls hooligan.*"

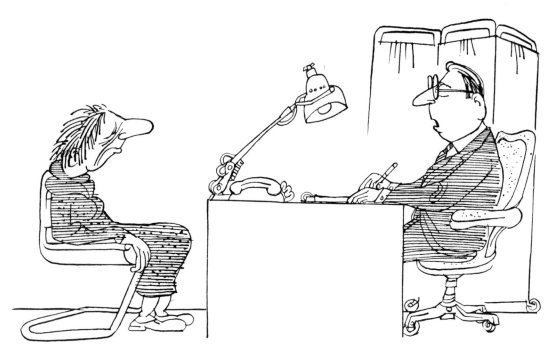

"Have you tried drink?"

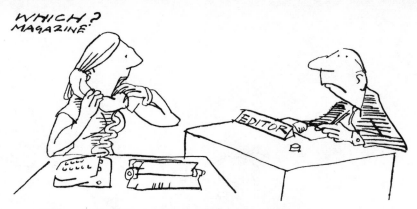

"*It's somebody complaining about the May issue.*"

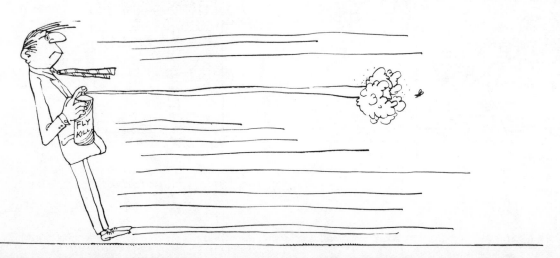

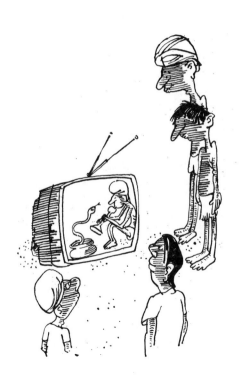

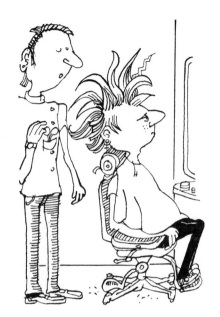

"Usual?"

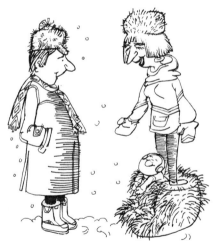

*"He's warm and it keeps him out
of mischief."*

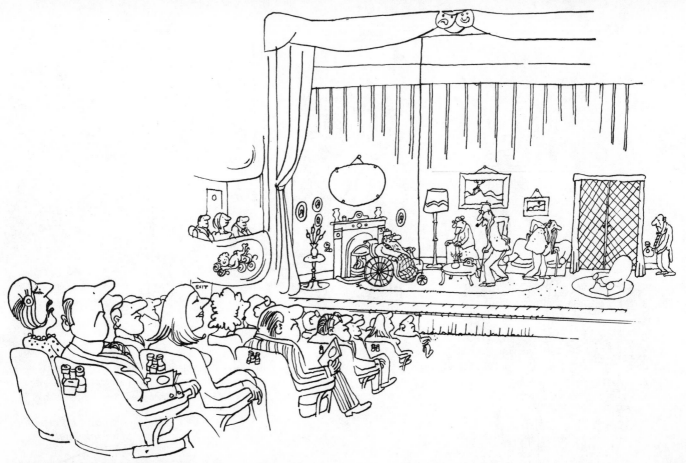

"Apparently it's had the longest run of any play in London."

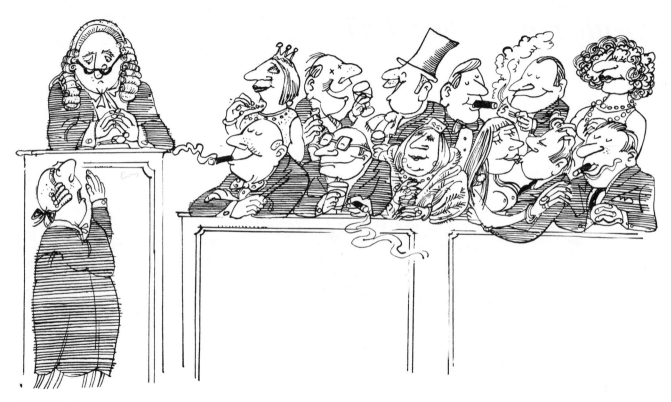

"*I think the jury has been got at, my lord.*"

Getting away from it all

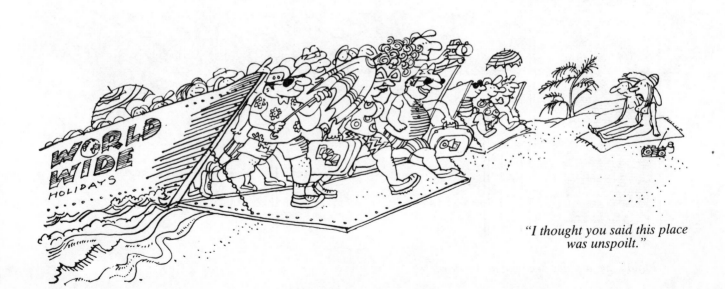

"*I thought you said this place was unspoilt.*"

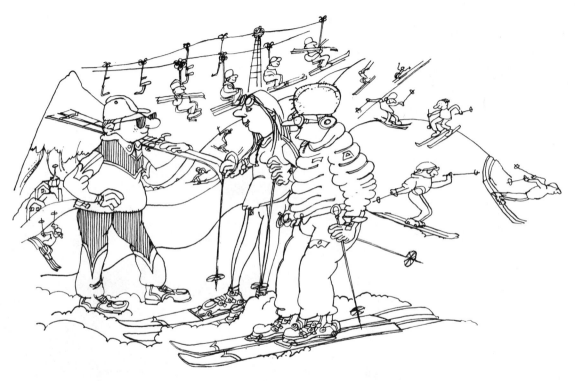

"We came here to get away from all those holiday
ads on television."

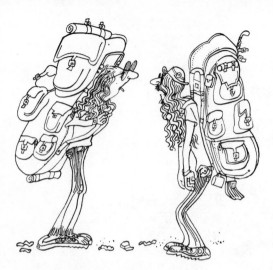

"I was wandering around mindlessly in New York, and I thought; why not wander around mindlessly in London?"

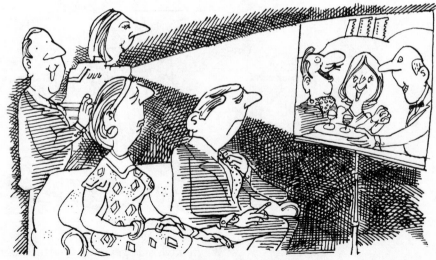

"We had a really awful holiday, so we borrowed these photographs from a couple who had a really good one."

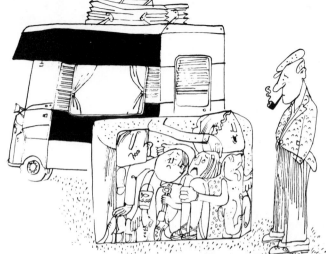

"*It was quite a squeeze but we had a great holiday.*"

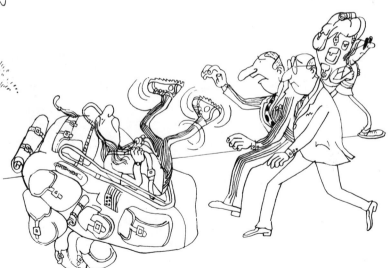

"*Apparently they die if they're not put the right way up.*"

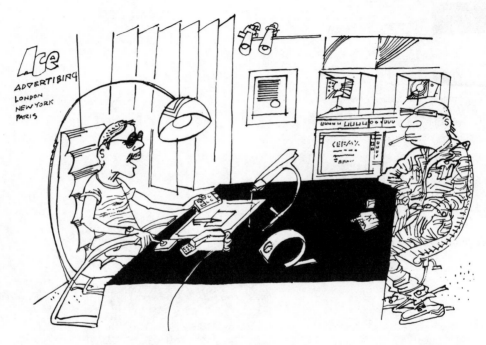

"*Your last commercial was great. Do you think you have enough suppressed genius to do another?*"

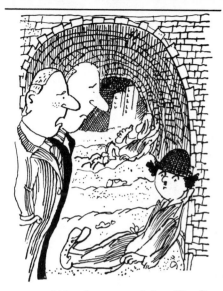

"It could be the memorial to Charlie Chaplin."

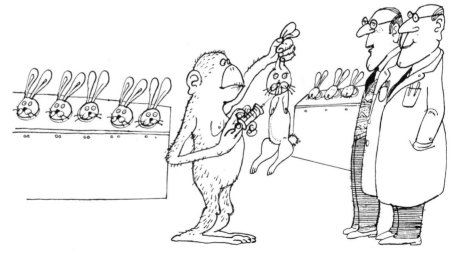

"Congratulations, Dr Weaser—you've trained him to be almost human."

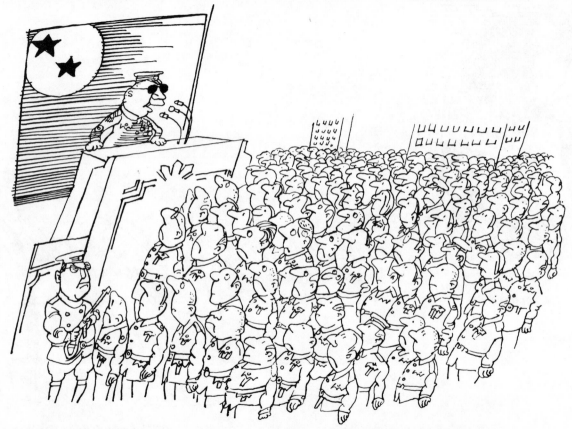

"So much for taking over the world—now I'd like to talk to you about double glazing..."

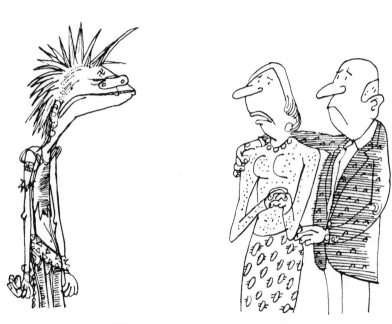

*"I know it's a bit late, but looking at our Nigel,
I think I'm starting a post-natal depression."*

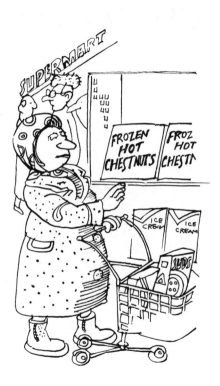

Christmas cheer

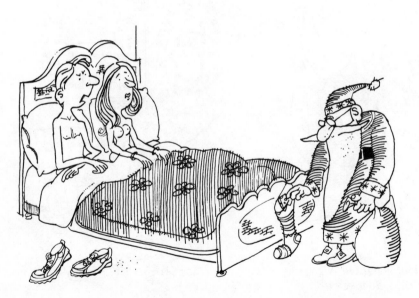

"It's only my father, he'll be gone in a minute."

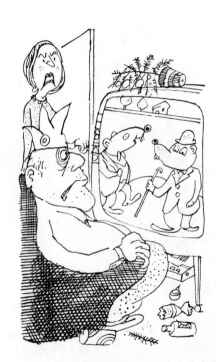

"You can turn it off now
Christmas is over."

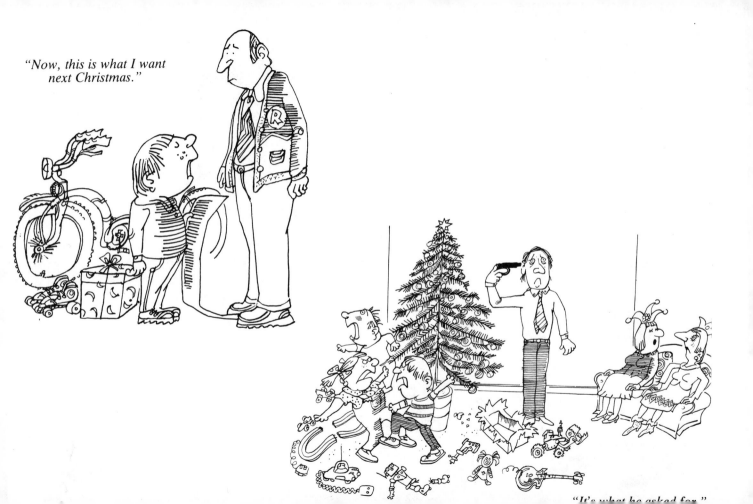

"Now, this is what I want next Christmas."

"It's what he asked for."

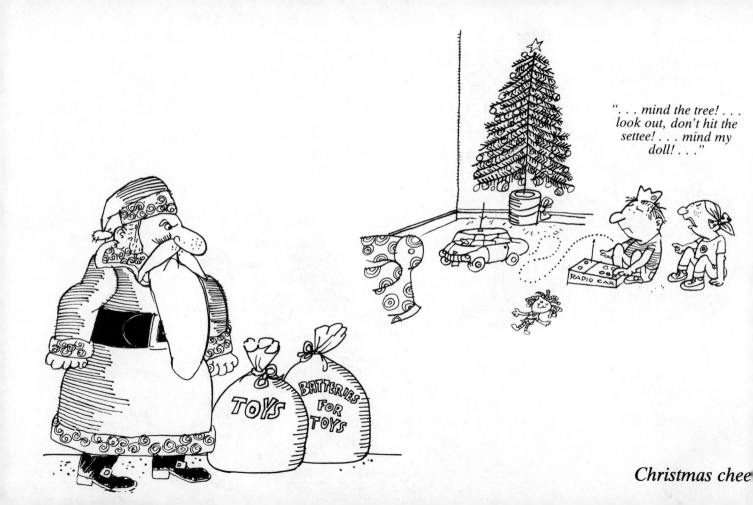

Christmas chee

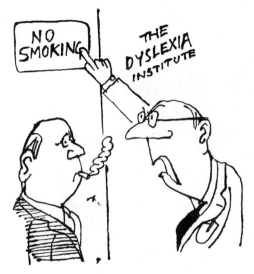

"Can't you read!"

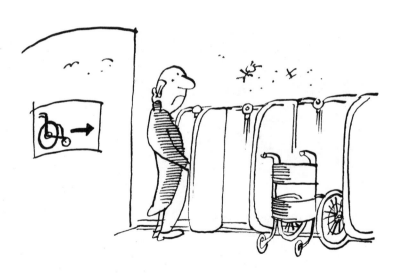

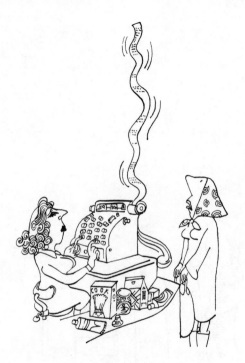

"I see the cost of living's going up again."

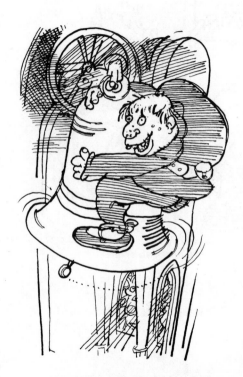

"At the third stroke it will be . . ."

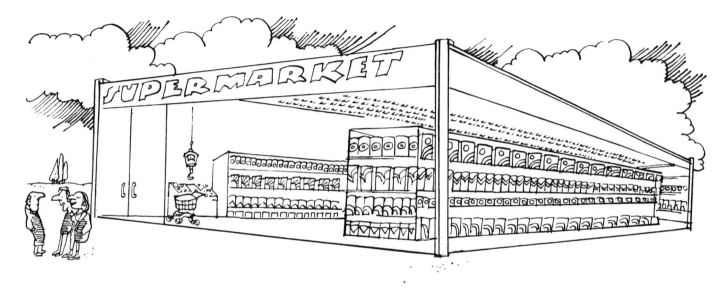

"It was Marjorie's idea to buy it. Now we're totally self-reliant."

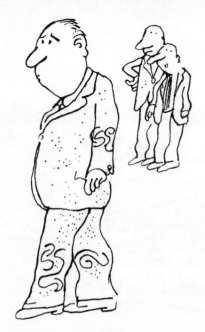

"In the 50s he modelled himself on James Dean, now it's Frank Bough."

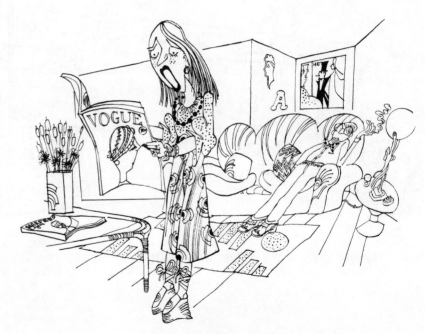

"My God! I've got last year's body!"

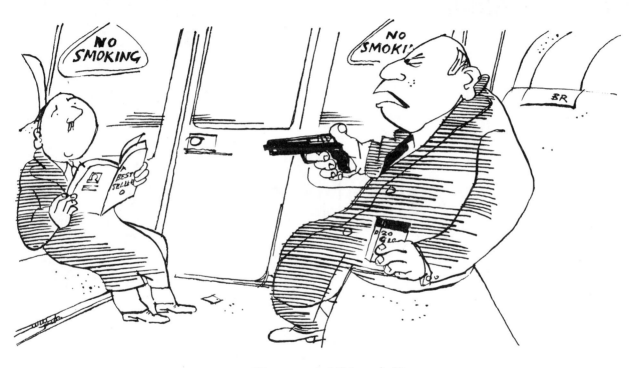

"Do you mind if I smoke?"

The Generations

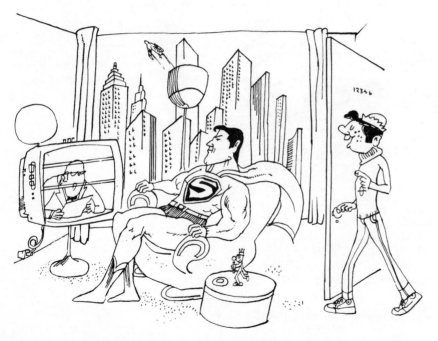

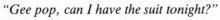

"Gee pop, can I have the suit tonight?"

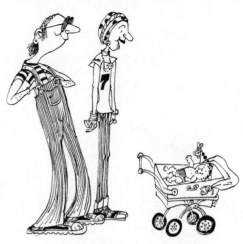

"I've made him some blue denim nappies."

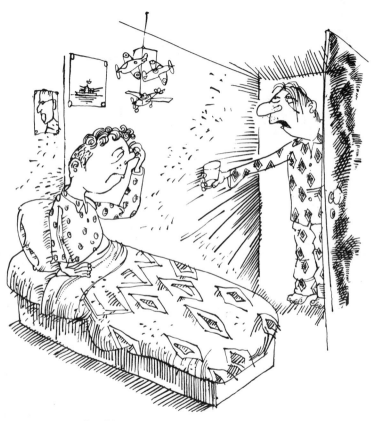

"Could you get me a glass of whisky?"

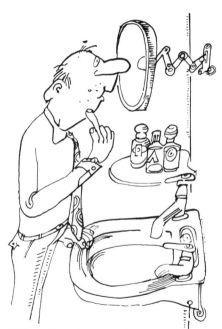

"That diet of jam and sweets is working! I'm getting acne!"

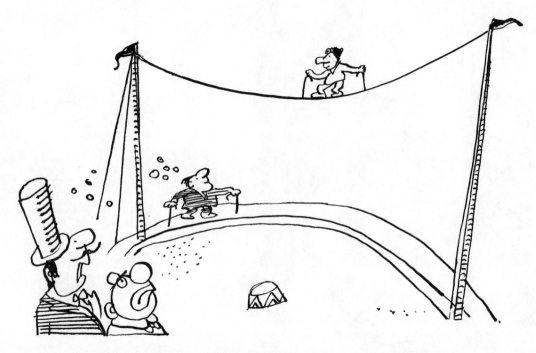

"After the Great Gramildi had that terrible fall,
he taught the kid everything he knew."

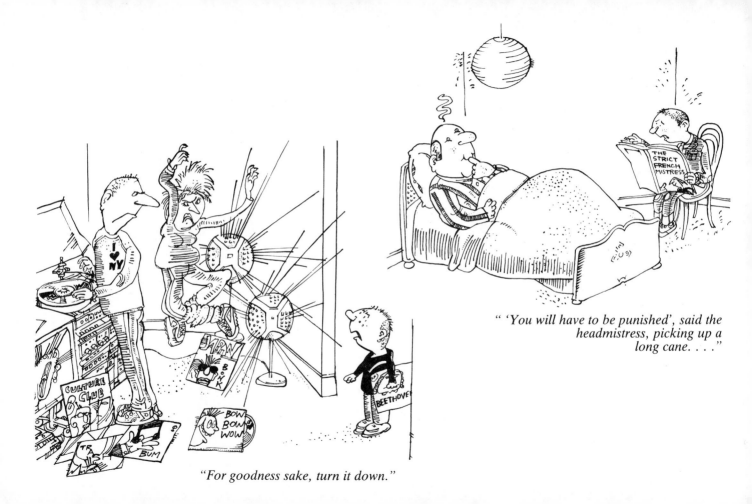

"For goodness sake, turn it down."

" 'You will have to be punished', said the headmistress, picking up a long cane. . . ."

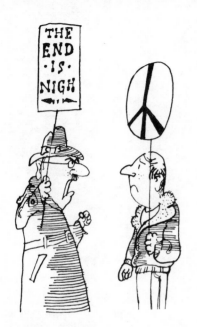

"I'm ashamed to be your father!"

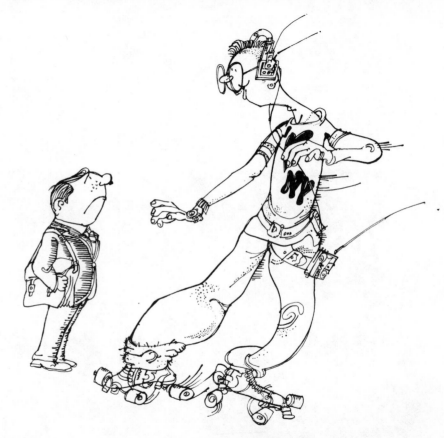

"I bet you can't wait to grow up, son!"

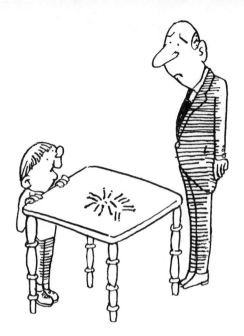

"Look, Dad, I've made the Mary
Rose out of matches."

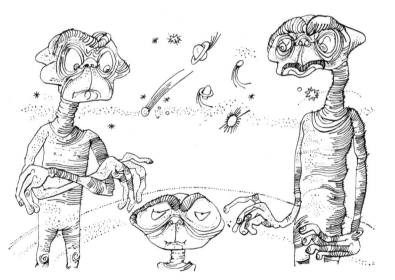

"Kids today! All they want to do, is go to
Earth and become film stars!"

The Generations

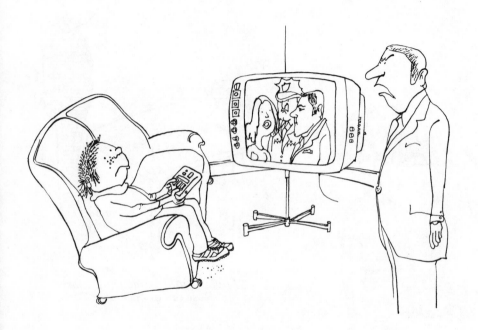

"When I was a boy, we used to make our own entertainment, like switching channels manually."

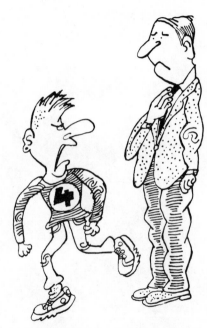

"What do you know about life—you're too old!"

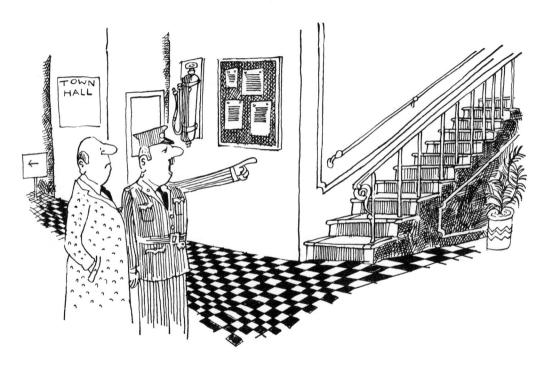

"*The city planning exhibition, yes, sir, up the stairs, turn left, and go down the corridor through the door marked exit and down the fire escape, across the yard . . .*"

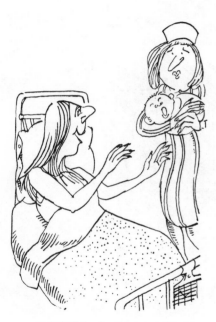

"Will he be a success?"

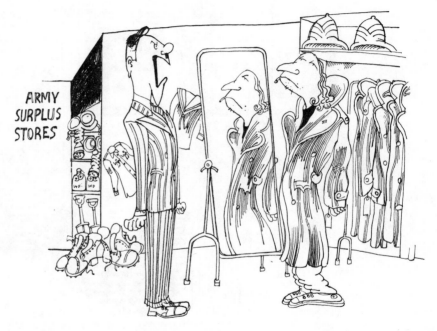

"Put your shoulders back, you horrible little man—Get your hair cut—
Pull yourself together, you pansy!"

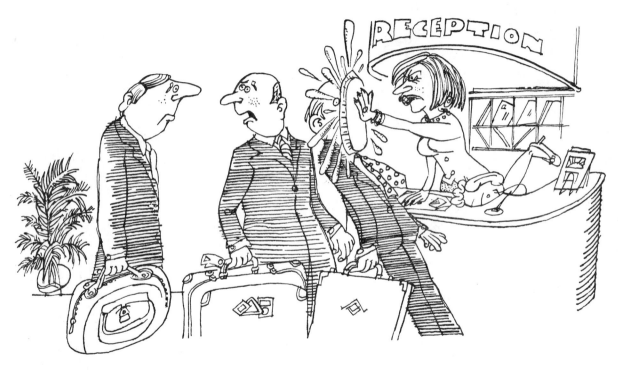

"*They're really tough here if they find you've exceeded your credit card limit.*"

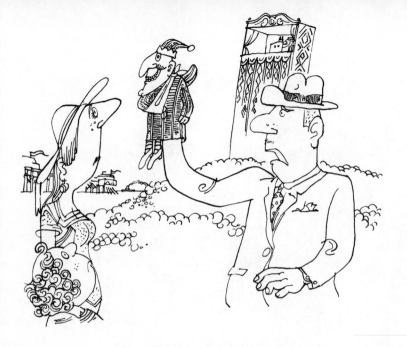

"There'll be no show today—I've broken my finger."

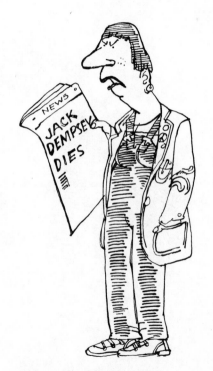

"I knew boxing was dangerous."

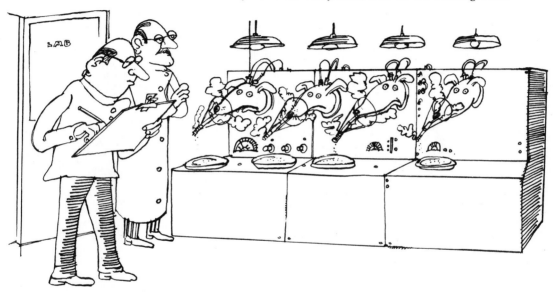

"*If we're his best friend, how do the others get on?*"

Doctors and patients

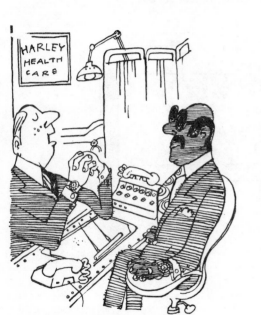

"*Or for a little extra you can have the 'Gucci' heart.*"

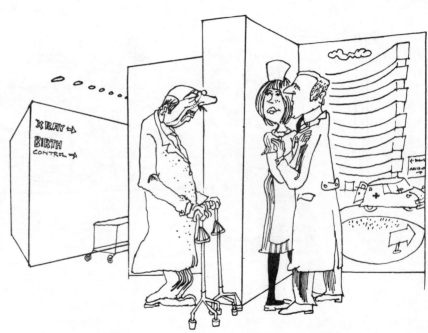

"*Would you be the physiotherapist?*"

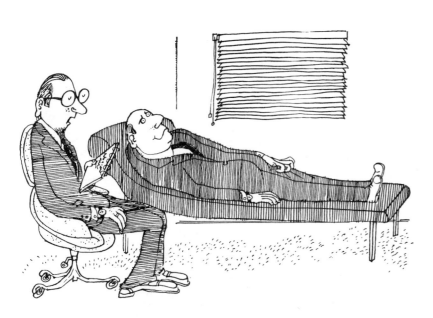

"Your sexual desires are so odd that I suggest you start demonstrating for your rights immediately."

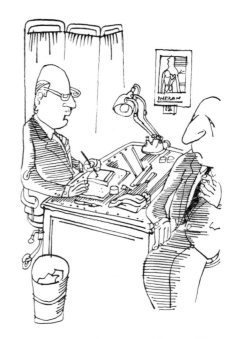

"I want you to take these tablets and lay off trying to keep fit for a while."

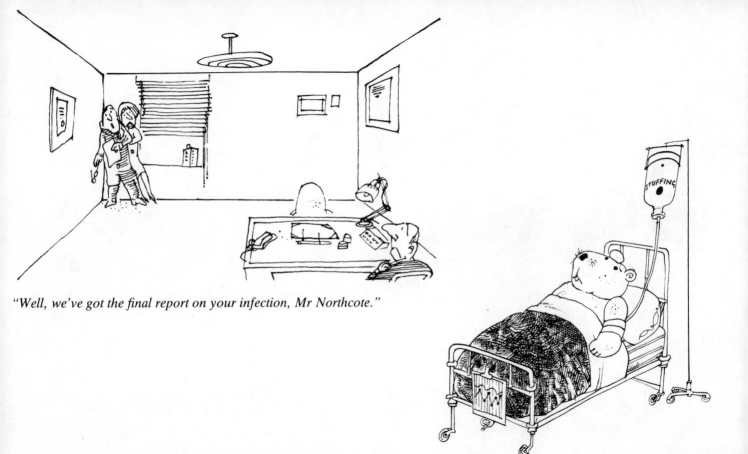

"*Well, we've got the final report on your infection, Mr Northcote.*"

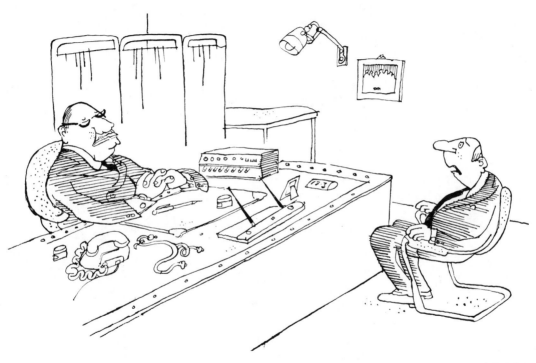

"Give it to me straight, doctor—is what I've got worth televising?"

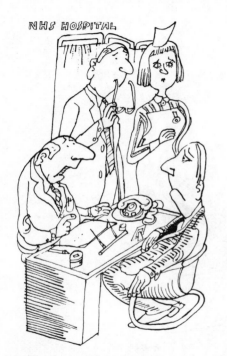

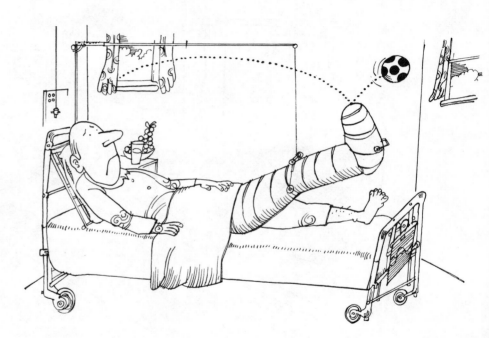

"Well, yes, you are an emergency. We'd like to operate this afternoon. Could you go home and get your night things, and on your way back could you buy a scalpel and some antiseptic and don't forget some bandages!"

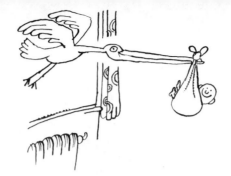

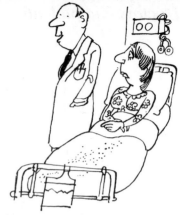

"We still believe that the old methods
are best Mrs Simmonds."

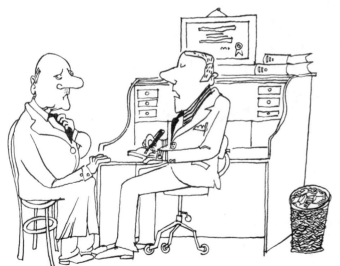

"There's nothing much wrong with you, it's just
that you're becoming obsolete."

Doctors and patients

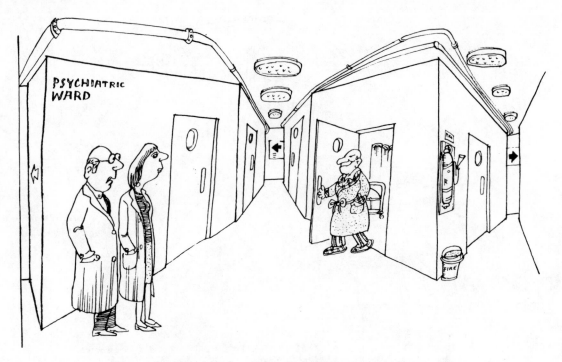

"I'm rather worried about him. He's beginning to adjust to the outside world."

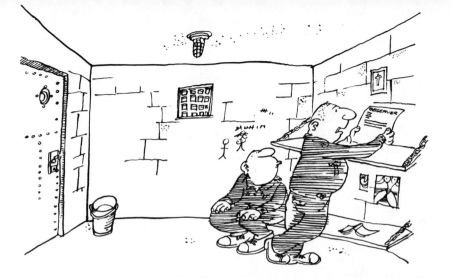

"It's from 'The Observer', they want me to
talk about my room."

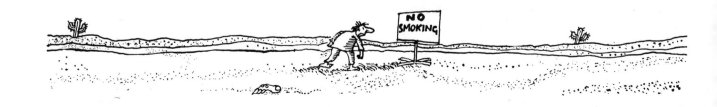

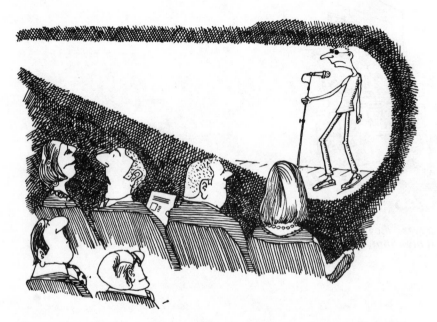

"It says here that he's a new comedian, and he hopes that we will find his material very offensive."

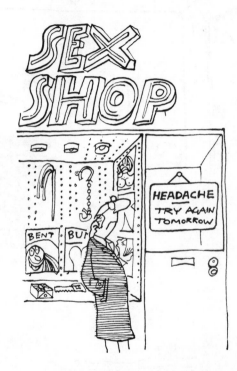

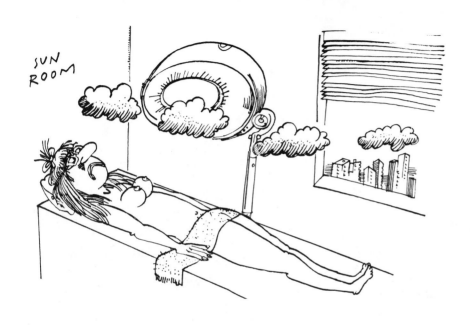

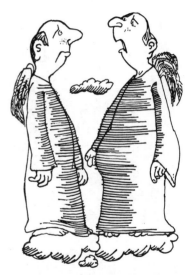

"I drank myself to death—now I'm rather lost for anything to do."

The Media

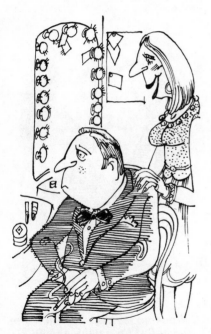

"Don't be so depressed—someone came to see us last night and she liked it."

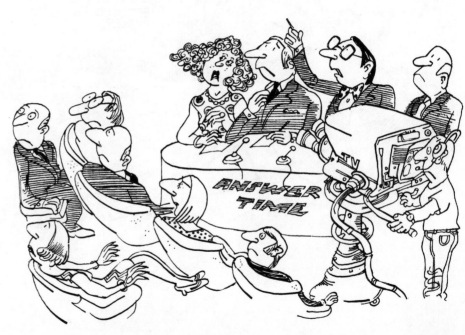

"Er . . . the woman at the back with the bomb in her hand . . ."

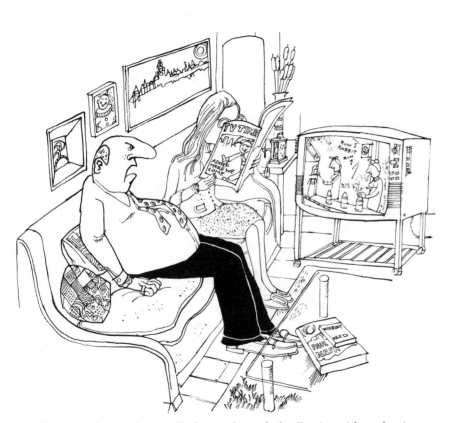

"It was bad enough actually living through the Forties without having to do it all over again!"

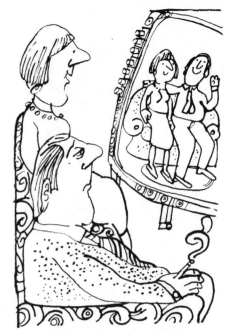

"Oh, look, it's the people next door—they must have got their own television show."

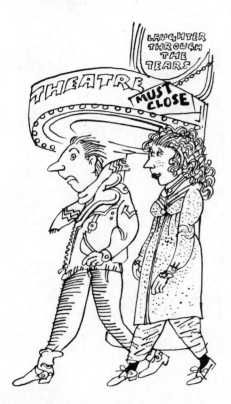

"*I don't know why it's coming off—it got lousy reviews.*"

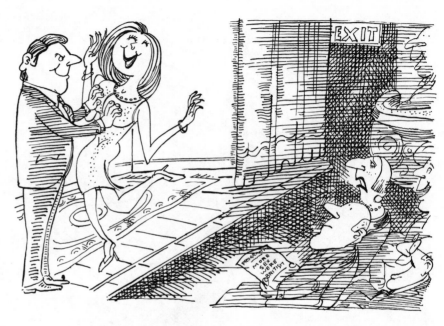

"*In my day, actors didn't know what to do with their hands!*"

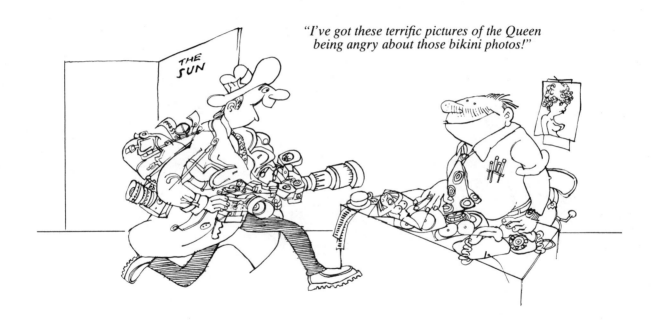

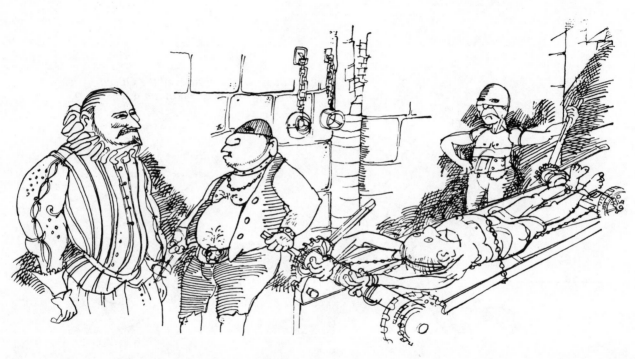

"This is John Smyth, he's a catholic, and he's going to answer questions on his specialist subject, priest holes in the Midlands."

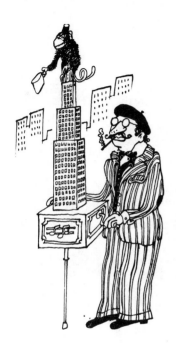

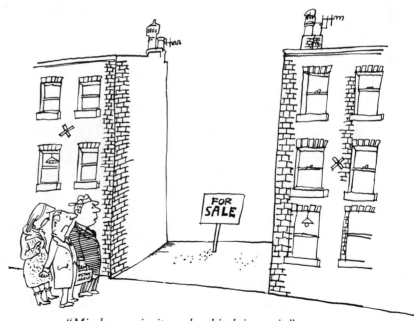

"Mind you, sir, it needs a bit doing to it."

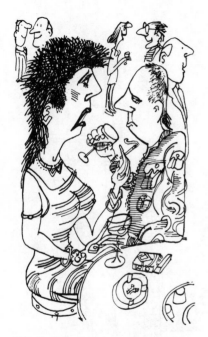

"Well, I don't know why you're so unhappy—it's not as if you were famous or anything."

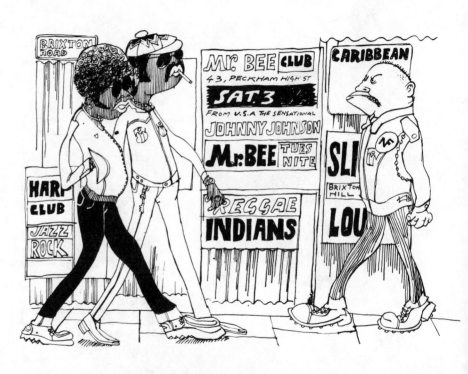

"I wouldn't like to meet him on a light night."

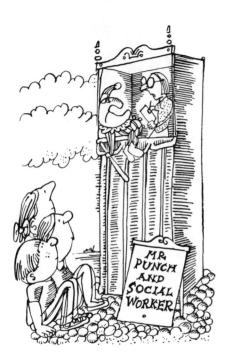

MR. PUNCH AND SOCIAL WORKER

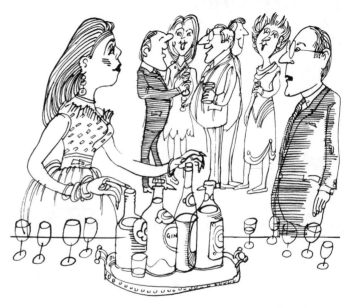

"I'm trying to give it up—have you got any glue?"

Funny valentines

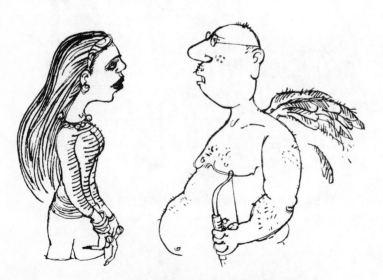

"Even cupids grow old, my dear."

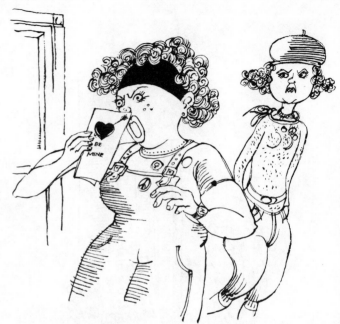

"You can tell it's from a man, it smells of perfume!"

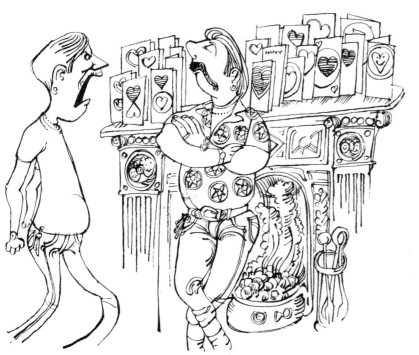

"*Well, 450 Valentine cards suggest promiscuity to me.*"

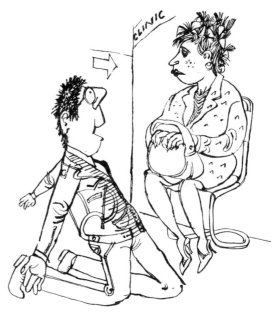

"*Marry me, Miss Baker—after all, we both have the same social disease.*"

Funny valentines

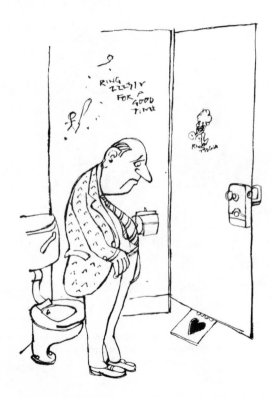

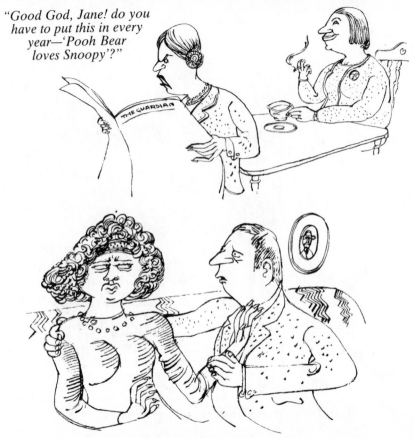

"*Good God, Jane! do you have to put this in every year—'Pooh Bear loves Snoopy'?*"

"*I hope you don't think I'm being sexist, Margery, but I love you!*"

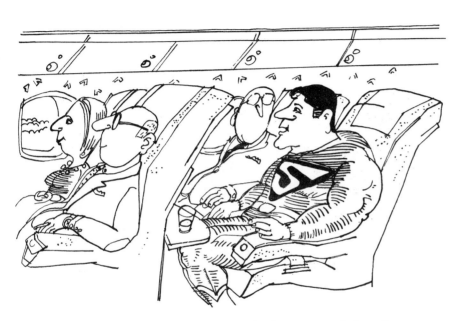

"Oh, I just got kinda fed up with the flying around alone."

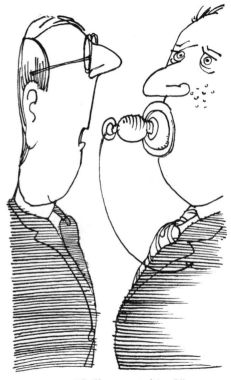

"Still not smoking?"

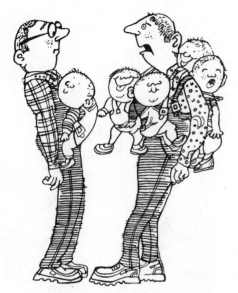

*"Of course, quads were quite a shock
at first."*

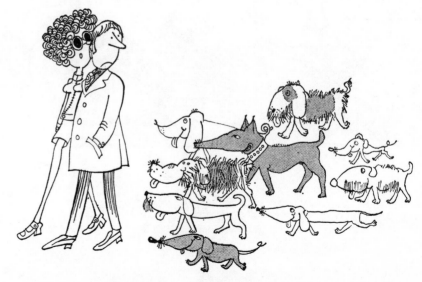

"You've overdone the aftershave again."

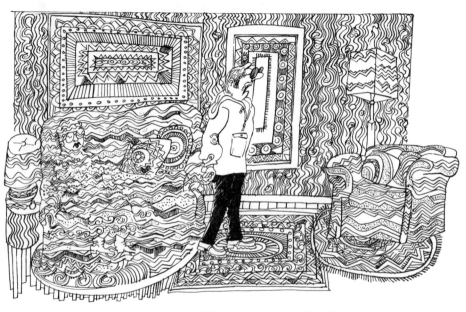

"Where are you darling?"

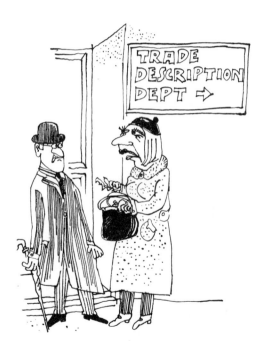

"Like to pay through the nose for a dreary time, dear?"

Streetwise

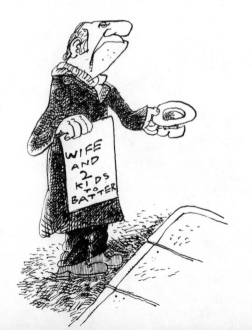

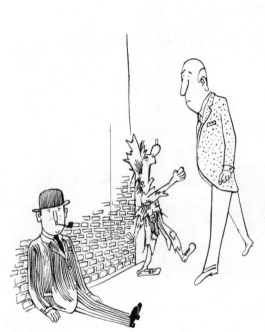

"*Penny for the guy!*"

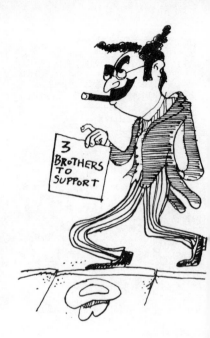

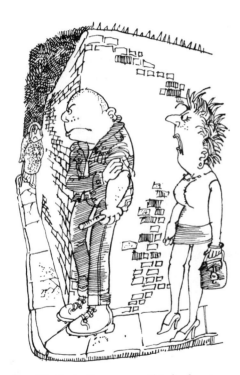

"Is that all you ever think about—
work?"

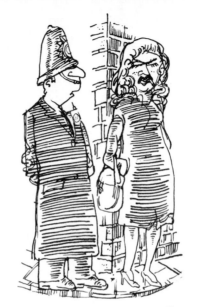

"Move along, Doreen, or I'm
goin' to have to put a clamp on you."

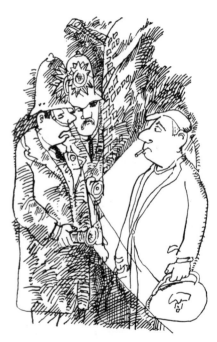

"OK, what's goin' on? And don't give
me that one about bein' a TV-am
newsreader."

Streetwise

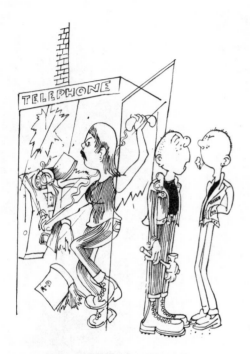

*"Have you noticed how long a
woman takes to vandalise a phone?"*

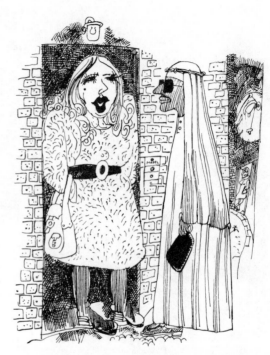

*"I can do the thou bit, but the jug of
wine and book of verse will cost you extra."*

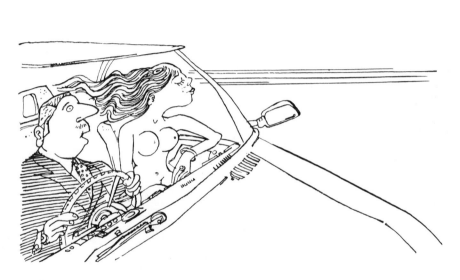

"I don't normally give lifts."

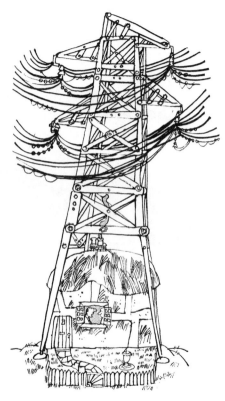

"I told them straight, I wasn't going to have their rotten old pylon ruining my view."

"Sorry, mate, I'm on my way back home to Clapham."

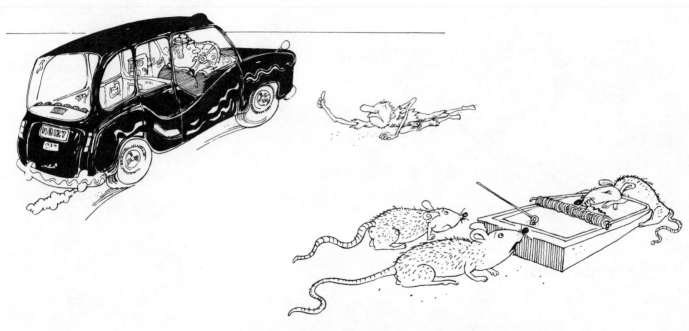

"I always did think those take-aways were bad for you."

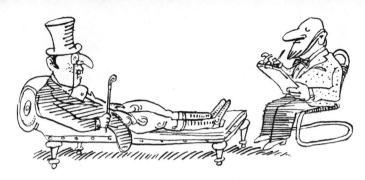

"I love killing foxes."

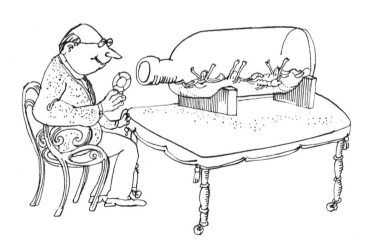

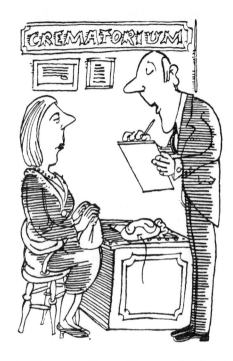

"And how would you like your husband
done, Mrs Wicks?"

The hard-up zoo

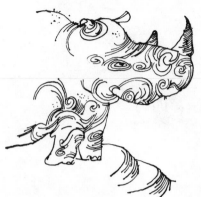

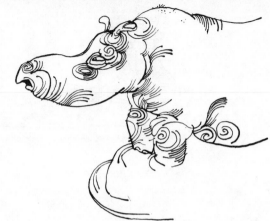

"I used to have a lovely horn but they sold it to a sex shop."

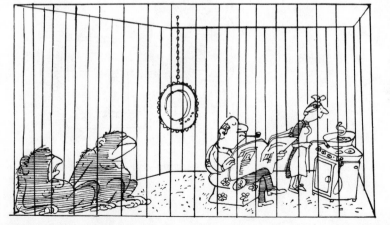

"I'm not sure I like this time-sharing."

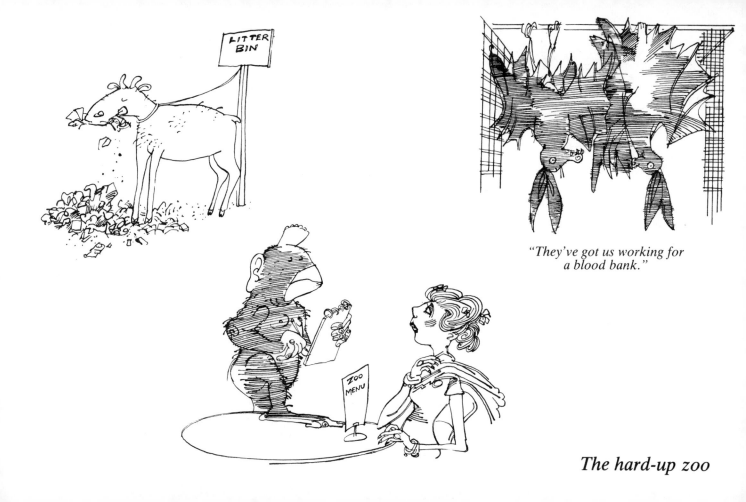

"They've got us working for
a blood bank."

The hard-up zoo

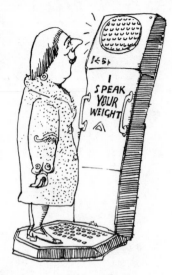

"You've lost seven pounds since you were last here—gosh, that's really terrific! What diet are you on—the Scarsdale? Yes, it seems to work really well on most people . . ."

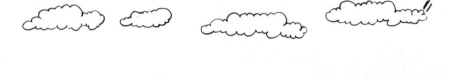

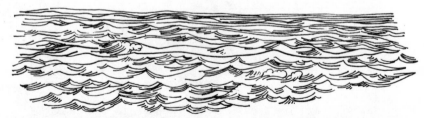

"The area we are passing over is commonly called the Bermuda Triangle."

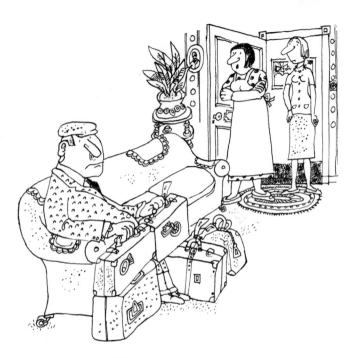

"He's never put down roots."

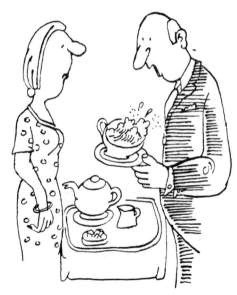

"Good Lord I never thought I'd live to see it, a storm in a teacup."

Kids of today

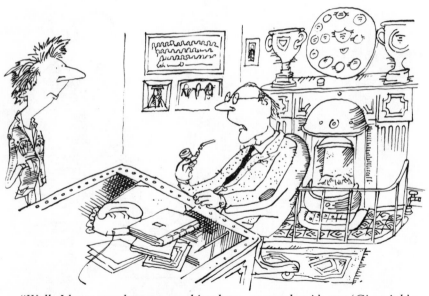

"Well, I hope you learnt something here—remember it's not 'Gissa job',
it's 'Have you any employment for me?'"

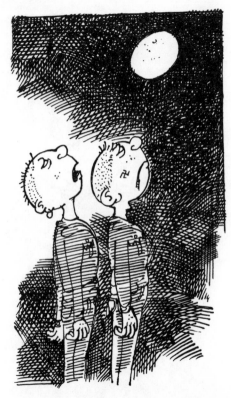

"I can't believe that there isn't another
planet out there with people as thick
as us on it."

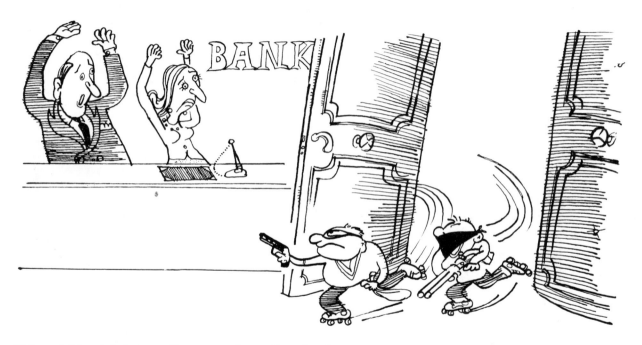

"I feared this might happen if we opened on a Saturday."

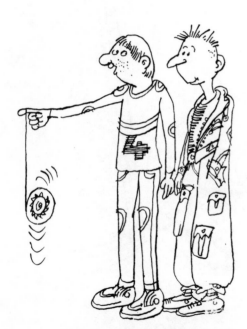

"It's electronic—it goes up and down without you doing anything."

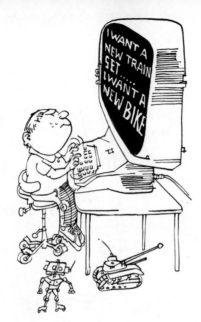

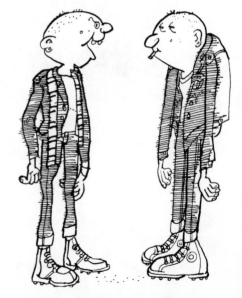

"I'm glad we can start bein' football hooligans again—I was gettin' fed up kickin' ol' ladies about."

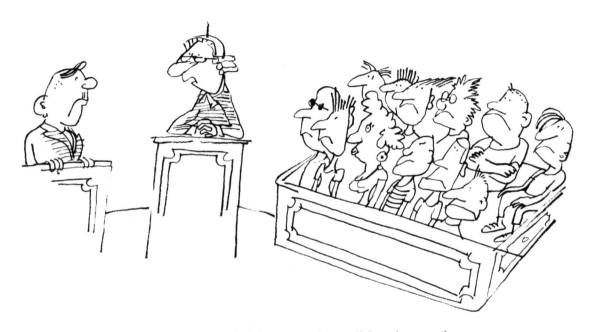

"These twelve wonderful teenagers have all found you guilty
of being fifty years old."

Kids of today

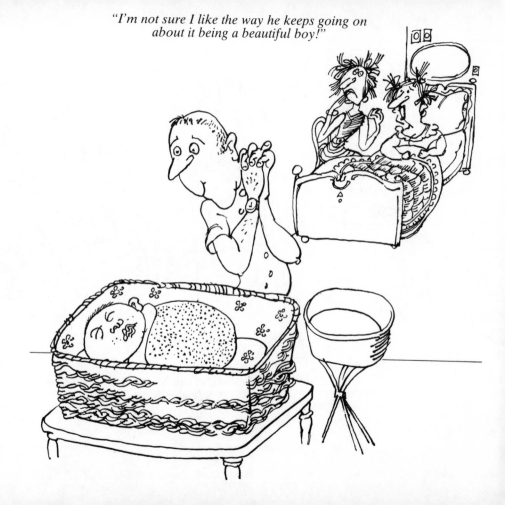

"I'm not sure I like the way he keeps going on about it being a beautiful boy!"

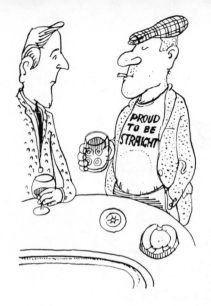

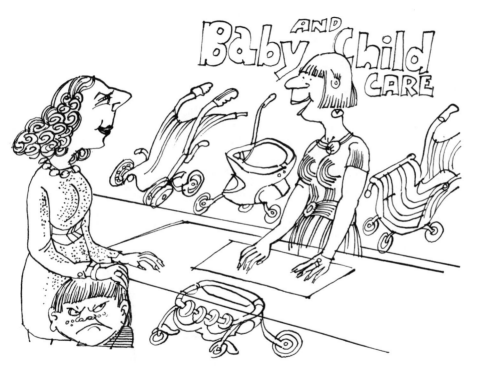

"*Corporal punishment? That's the fifth floor, madam.*"

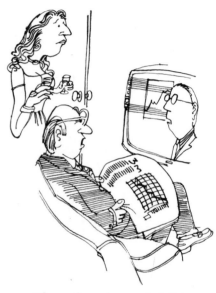

"*Soon the only people left in employment will be those writing and talking about it.*"

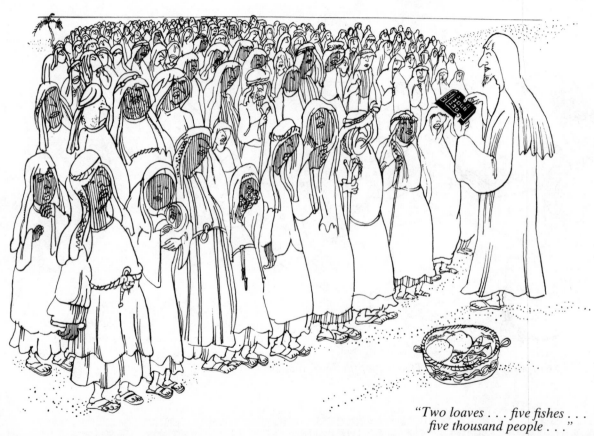

*"Two loaves . . . five fishes . . .
five thousand people . . ."*

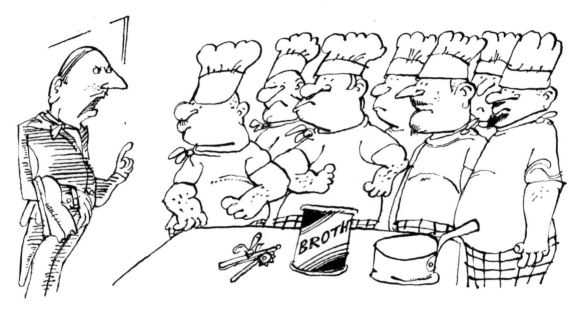

"Now whatever you do, don't spoil it!"

Animal ways

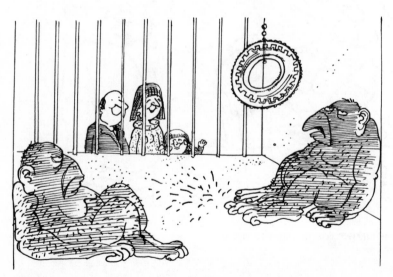

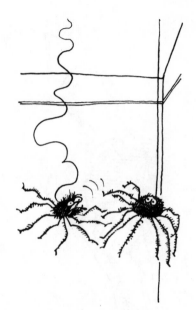

"With good behaviour you get to stay here for ever."

"I'm sorry—it's just that I've got this thing about spiders!"

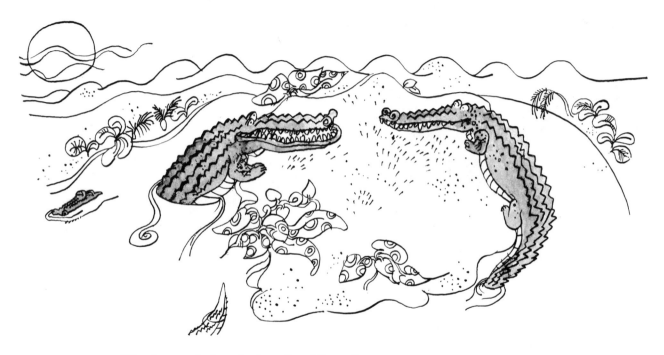

"I've bequeathed my body to Bond Street."

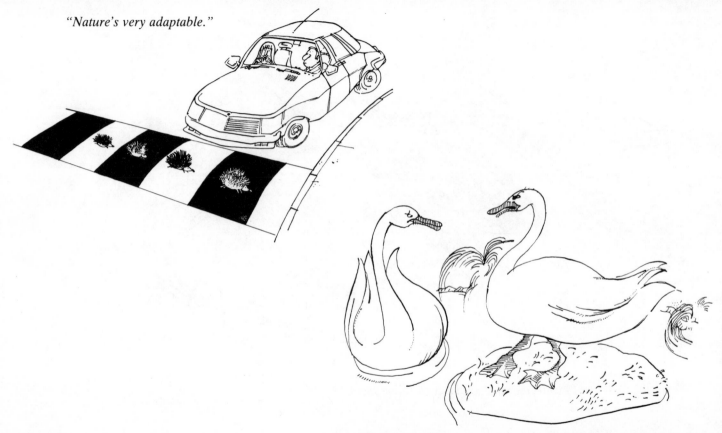

"Nature's very adaptable."

"You mean that now you've seen me walking, you don't find
me romantic anymore?"

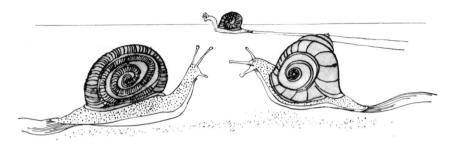

"He's such a snob he's changed his name to Escargot."

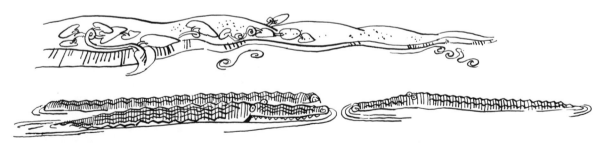

"You wouldn't have any trouble if you did what I did—I married a log."

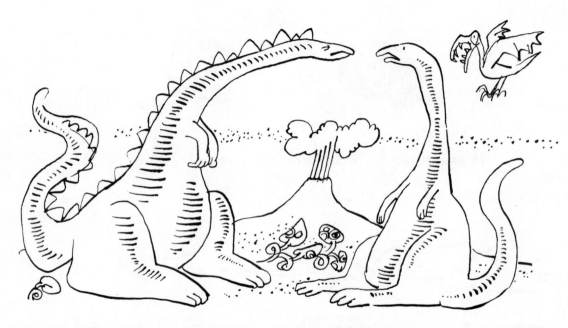

"*Of course you feel world weary, we all feel world weary at times.*"

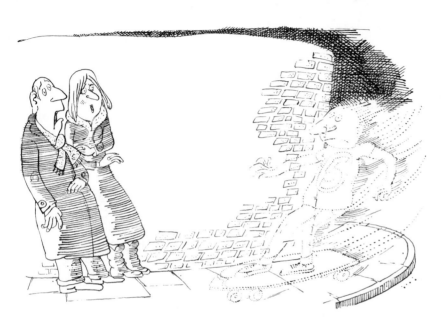

"It's just that one never thinks of new ghosts!"

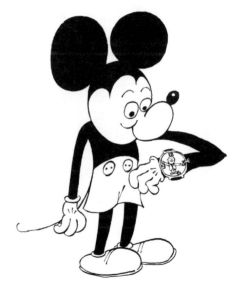

Law and order

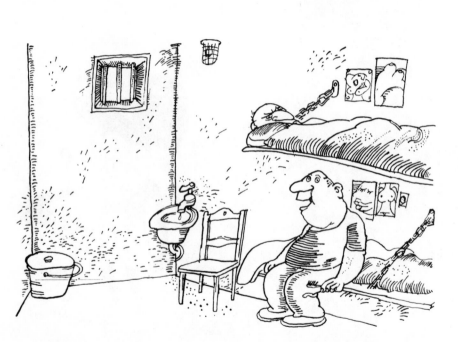

"It's Thursday, 6th August, 7 a.m. Good morning—it looks like it's going to be another warm day with temperatures in the eighties. I hope you have a nice day—your lucky star sign is Libra."

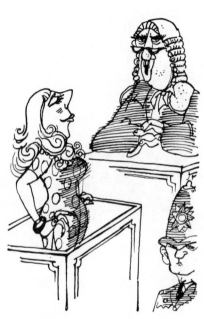

"You will be taken from here to a popular Sunday newspaper . . ."

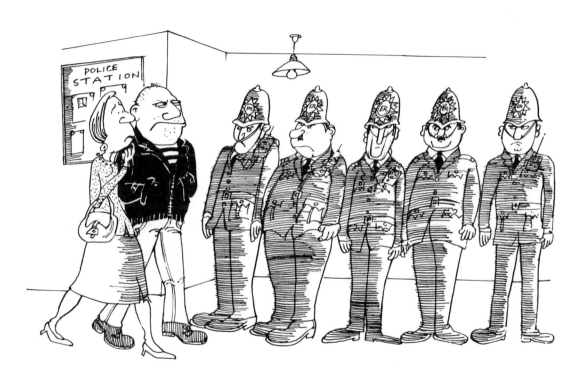

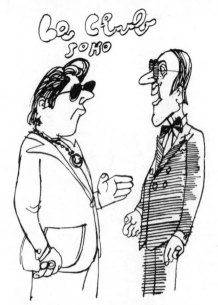

"How time flies! I remember when your father used to come round for the protection money."

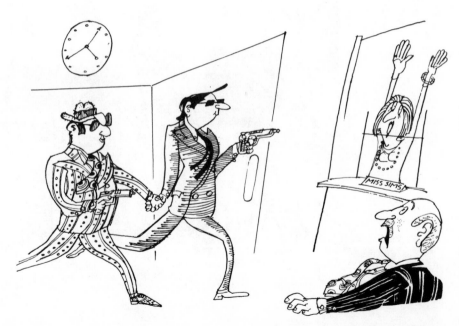

"Oh, my God! It's Clyde and Clyde!"

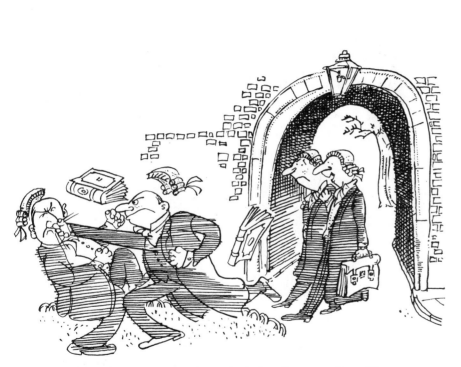

"I say, isn't that Owens v. Jones?"

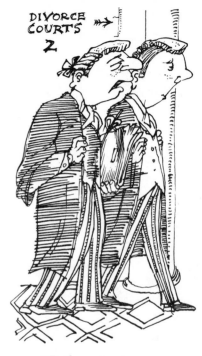

DIVORCE
COURTS →→
2

*"Rather a tragic case—
The Gambols."*

Law and order

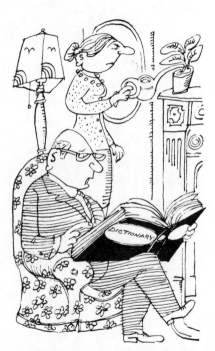

"That's odd, I can't find the word camouflage in here."

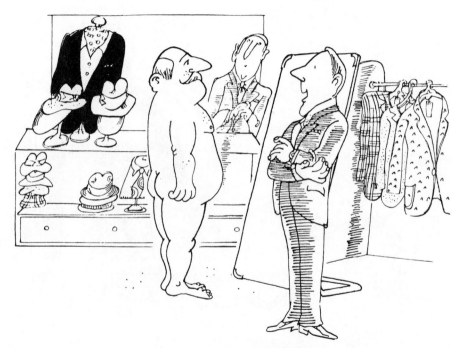

"It's what everyone's wearing in this hot weather, Your Majesty."

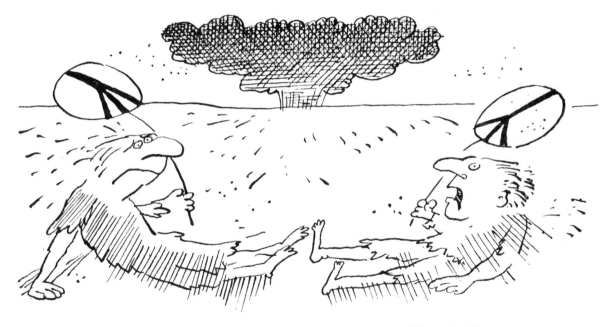

"Now what?"

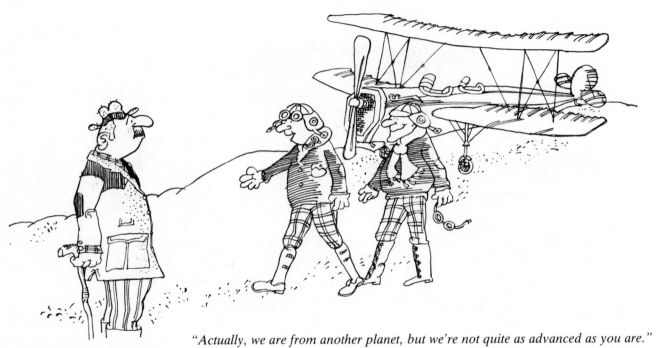

"*Actually, we are from another planet, but we're not quite as advanced as you are.*"

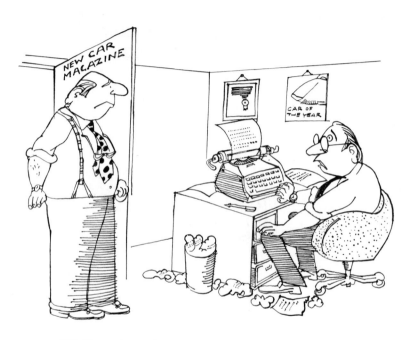

"Halfway through the article and I've run out of verbiage."

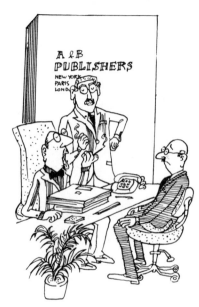

"Frankly, we like the book, but we don't think you're good-looking enough to sell it."

Low life

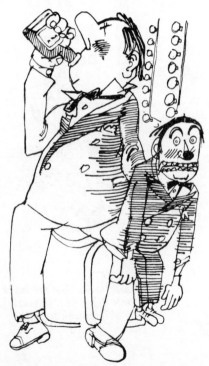

"Will someone take me away from him—he's turning me into a drunk!"

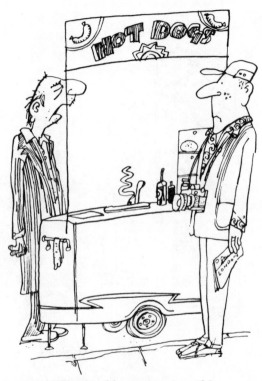

"They're fifty pee or sixty if I wash my hands."

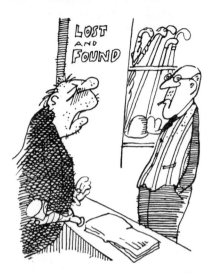

"I'm looking for last weekend."

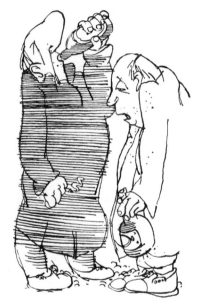

"In my case it all started with me trying to beat the Budget."

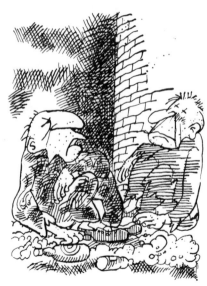

"Have you got a nail file?"

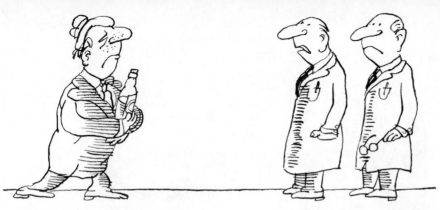

"We've got him off drinking but he won't let go of the bottle."

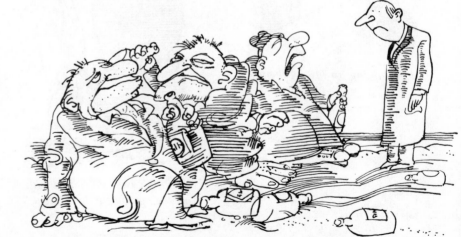

"We're all that's left of the Dean Martin Fan Club."

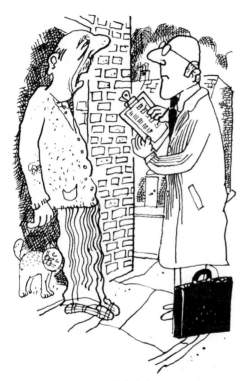

"If you people didn't keep coming round doing surveys on loneliness, I wouldn't see anyone."

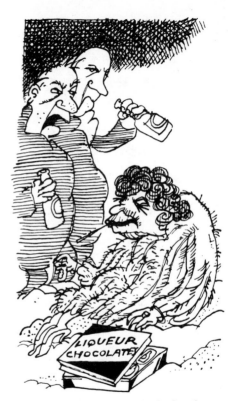

"She's much too la-di-da for the likes of us."

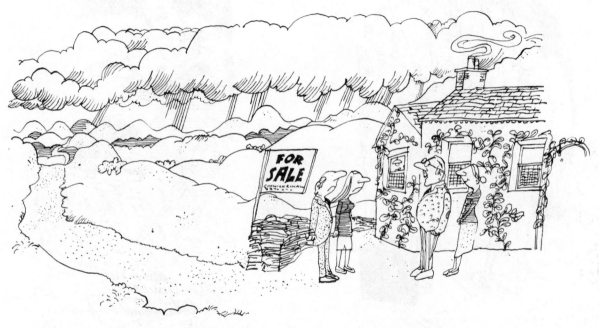

"It's not really for sale—we just don't see many people out here."

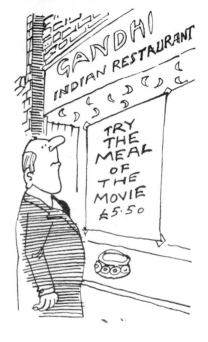
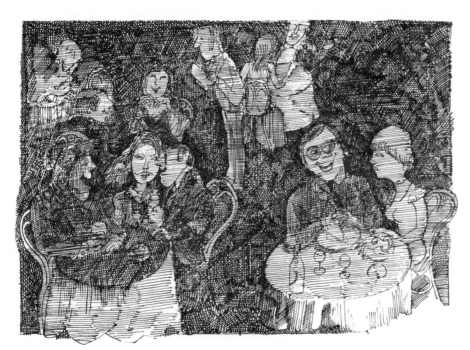

"Apparently this is the place to be seen in."

Christmas again

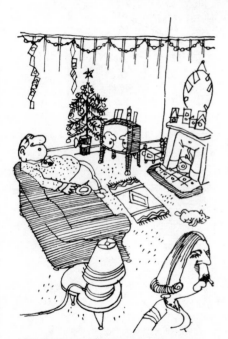

"Well, that's Christmas sorted out then—the first half of 'Gone with the Wind' here and the second half over at your Mother's on Boxing Day."

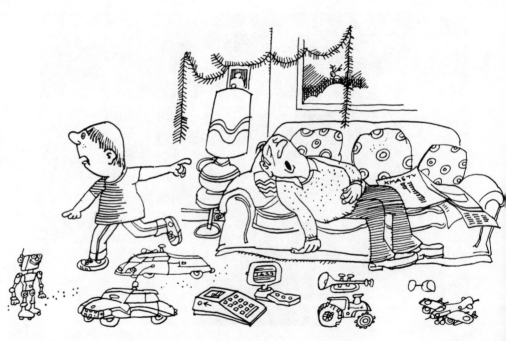

"Mummy! Mummy! Daddy's batteries have run out!"

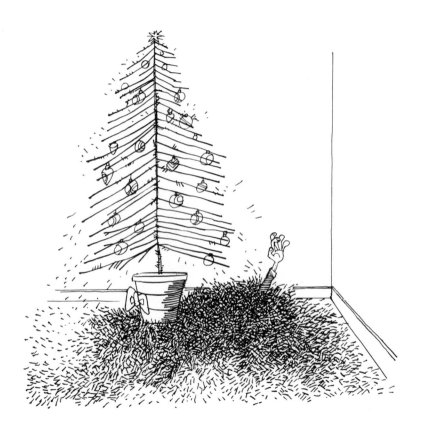

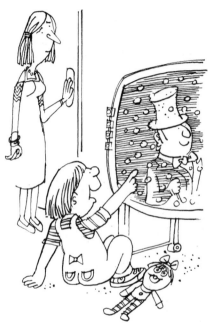

"Mummy! Mummy! It's snowing on television—I knew it would!"

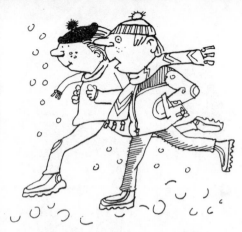

*"Quite a good Christmas, really—
my new Mum is much better than the
one Dad had last year."*

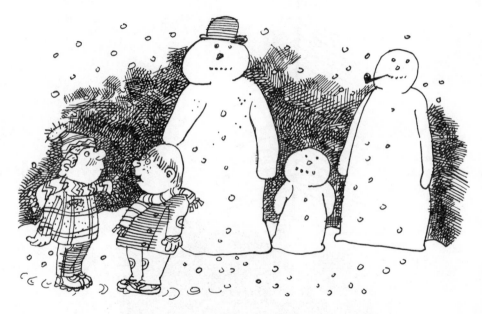

"It's a single-parent family and a social worker."

Christmas again

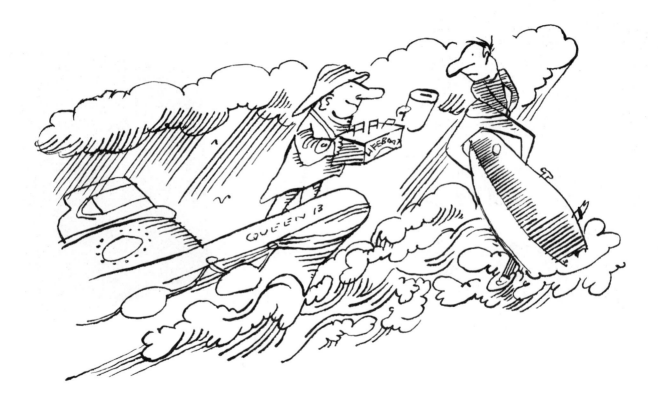

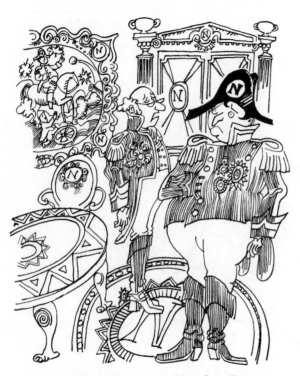

"But, sir, you are Napoleon!"

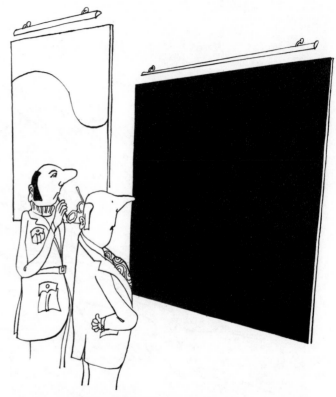

"How old hat it seems now."

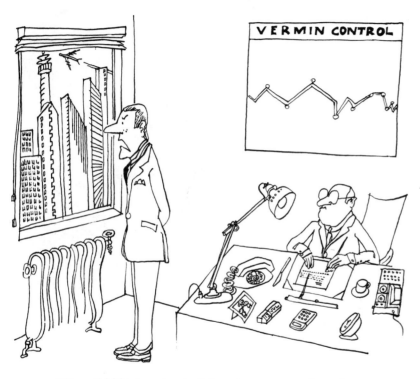

"How I'd like to get out of the rat, mouse, cockroach, silverfish, termite race."

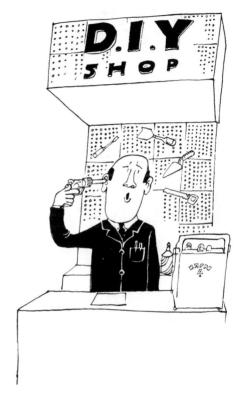

"O.K. fella! Hand over the money!"

Small talk

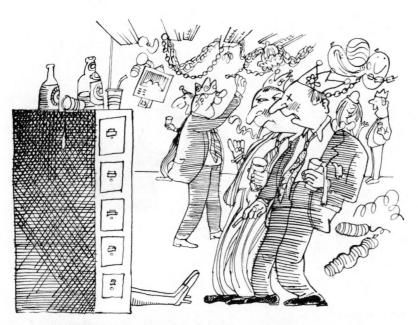

"She's either drunk, protesting against the bomb, or feeling sexy."

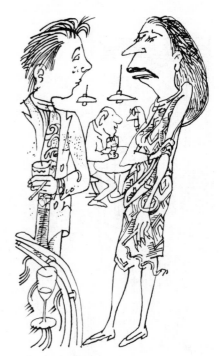

"I don't think they should bring back hanging—why don't they send them to live near army firing ranges?"

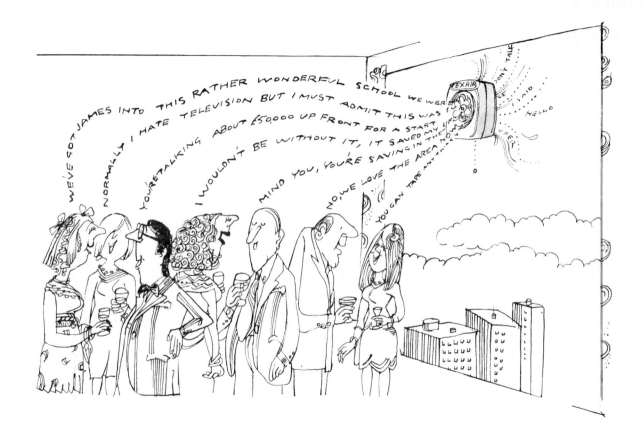

Small talk

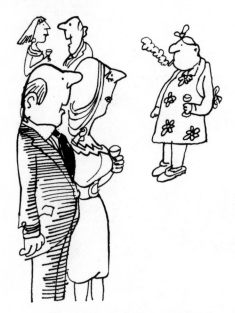

"Didn't he write all those kitchen sink dramas in the Fifties?"

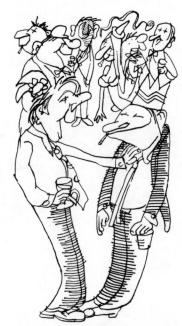

"Are you at my party enjoying yourself or am I at your party having a hell of a time?"

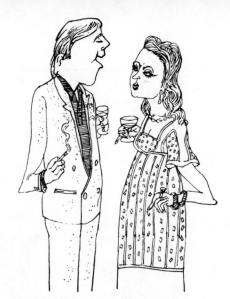

"I could be witty and erudite but I'm saving that up for my new talk show that starts this week."

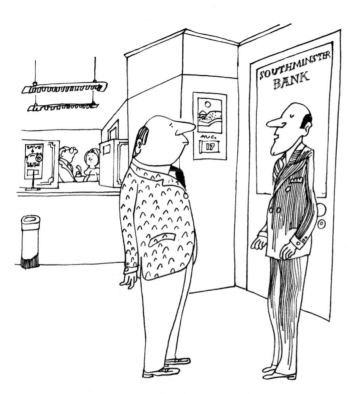

"I used to be an artist but I ran away
to become a bank manager."

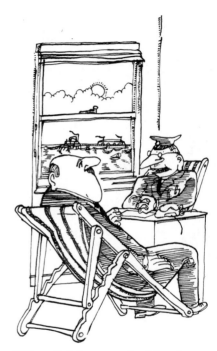

"We at Brightsea are looking for a top
deckchair attendant with experience.
Are you that man?"

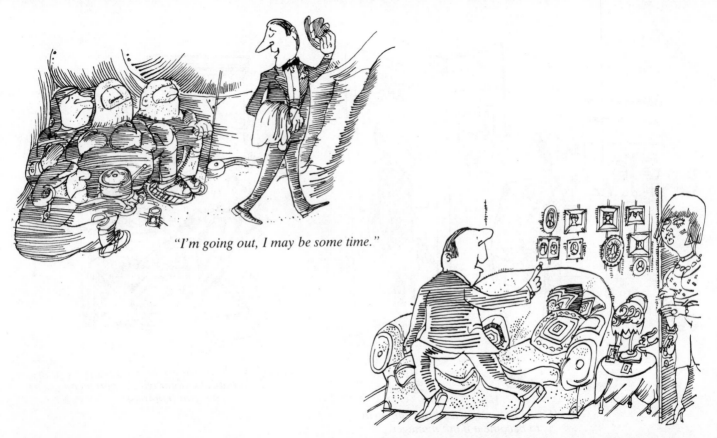

"I'm going out, I may be some time."

"I can't find the telly, but I have found your contact lens."

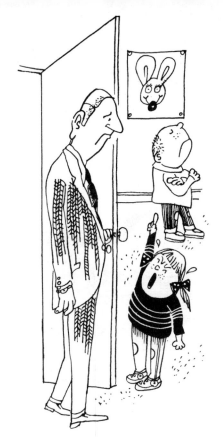

"We were playing Mummies and
Daddies and he refuses to pay me
alimony!"

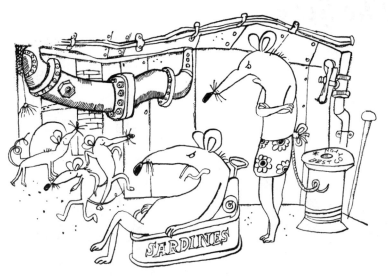

"Now if you were Mighty Mouse we wouldn't be stuck down
here in this lousy hole."

The Sexes

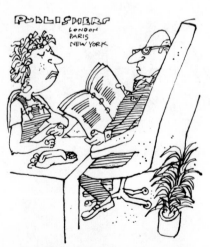

"You should have brought it to me last year—we were buying any book written by a woman then."

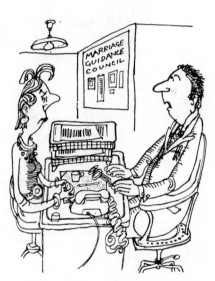

"I've asked you here because I want a divorce."

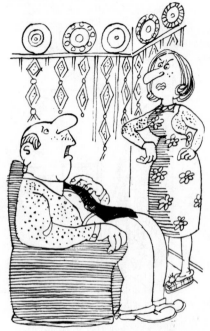

"I was just wondering if you'd be better or worse as a feminist."

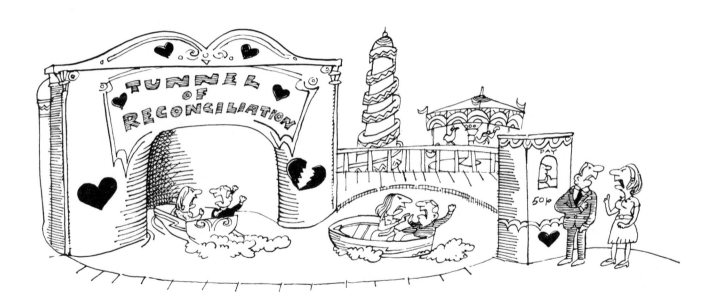

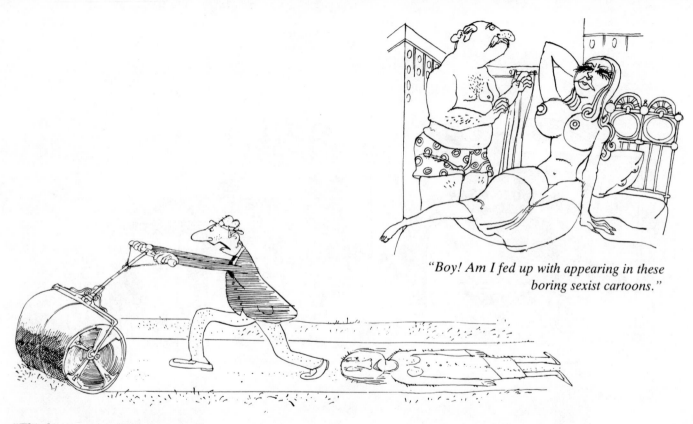

"Boy! Am I fed up with appearing in these boring sexist cartoons."

"This lawn gets worse every year!"

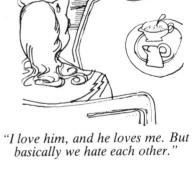

"I love him, and he loves me. But basically we hate each other."

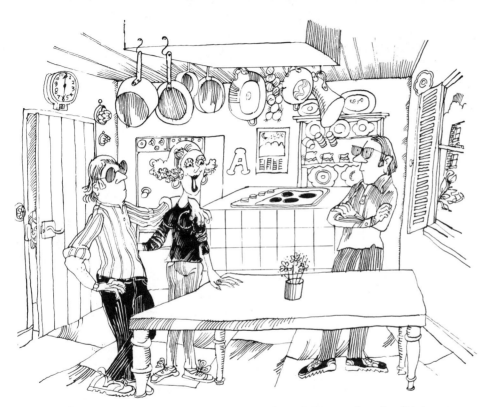

"Trevor went and bought this super table with his own hands, didn't you, Trevor?"

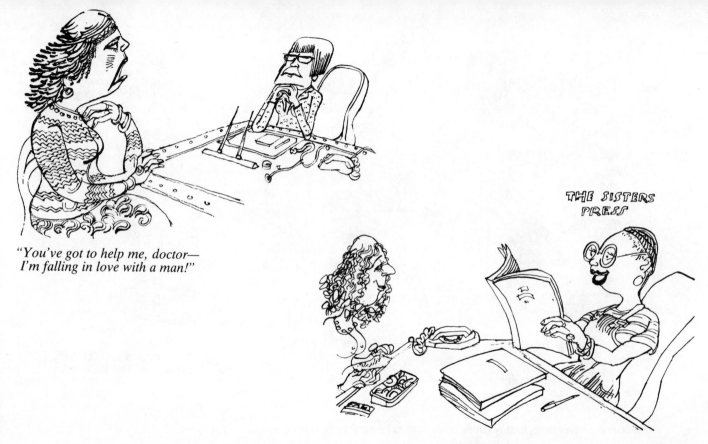

THE SISTERS PRESS

"You've got to help me, doctor—
I'm falling in love with a man!"

" 'Three Women in a Boat'—I like it!"

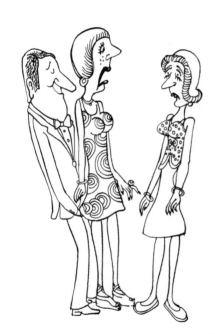

"He says he works on The Muppets."

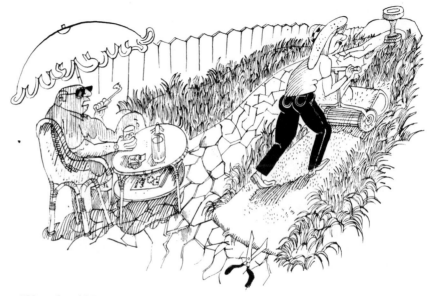

"You should have nagged at me for several weeks, I might have done it."

The Sexes

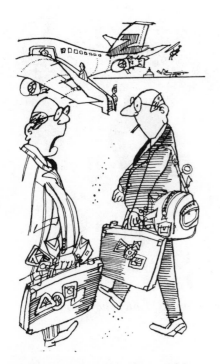

"When I was young, they said I was going places, but I never realised how awful these places were going to be."

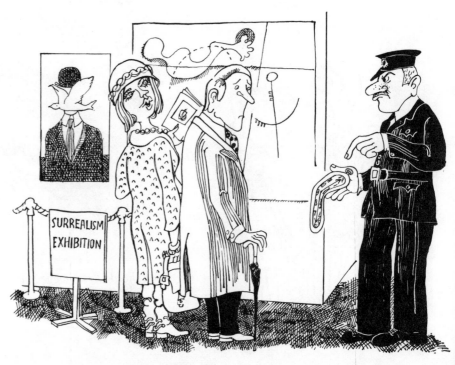

SURREALISM EXHIBITION

"I think he's trying to tell us they're closing."

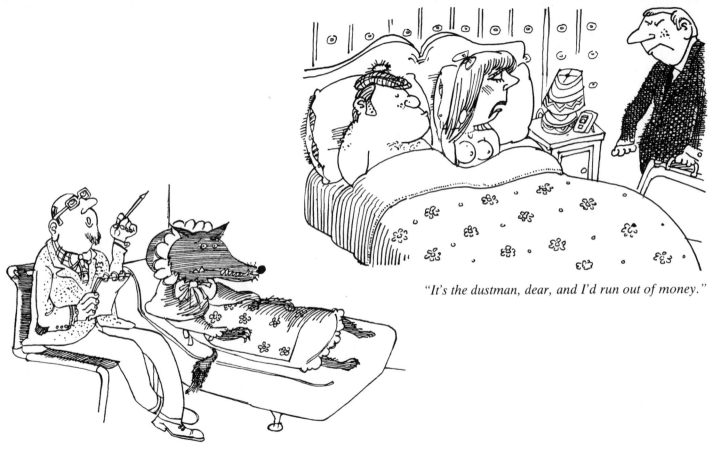

"It's the dustman, dear, and I'd run out of money."

"When did you first feel the need to wear women's clothing?"

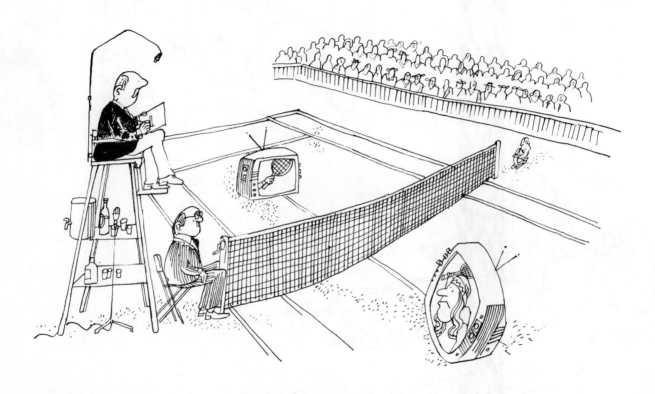